# DEAFNESS

# DEAFNESS

by Jane Hyman

A GROLIER COMPANY

FRANKLIN WATTS
NEW YORK | LONDON | TORONTO | SYDNEY | 1980
A FIRST BOOK

TO STEVEN, MICHAEL, AND WENDY

The author would like to thank Dr. Penny Axelrod
for her excellent comments and suggestions
concerning the manuscript for this book.

Diagrams by Vantage Art, Inc.

Photographs courtesy of: Wide World Photos:
pp. 4, 25, 50; Lexington School for the Deaf, New
York City: pp. 17, 20, 45; United Press Interna-
tional: pp. 37, 42; David Havs/The National Theatre
of the Deaf: p. 30.

Library of Congress Cataloging in Publication Data

Hyman, Jane.
    Deafness.

    (A First book)
    Bibliography: p.
    Includes index.
    SUMMARY: Discusses types of hearing losses
and their causes, the effects of deafness on the
individual, methods of learning speech and language, and alternative forms of communication.
    1. Children, Deaf—Juvenile literature.  2.
Deafness—Juvenile literature. [1. Deaf.  2. Phys-
ically handicapped]  I. Title.
RF291.5.C45H94      618.92'0978      80–15676
ISBN 0–531–02940–9

# Contents

# DEAFNESS

# Chapter 1
# "SOMETHING IS WRONG WITH CHRISTOPHER, DOCTOR"

Friday was a pleasant sunny day. Beth and Susan were waiting for their parents to bring home their new baby brother. At last, the car pulled into the driveway. Mrs. Stone brought Christopher into the house and put him in his crib to nap. Everything seemed just fine.

During his first few months of life, Chris behaved like almost any other baby. He ate and slept most of the time. He cried when he was hungry and when he was wet. Mrs. Stone brought him to the doctor's office for his regular checkups, and nothing special was ever said.

When Chris was several months old, however, Mrs. Stone began to worry. Something wasn't exactly right. Chris really didn't show much interest in speech or other sounds. His

[1

mother's voice did not seem to make him happy. He made sounds by himself, but Chris didn't show any interest in his musical toys unless he could see them. Loud noises did not surprise him. By the time Chris began to crawl, Mrs. Stone was very upset. "No, Chris," she would say, but Chris didn't seem to stop or listen unless he could see her. It was time to have a talk with the doctor.

Mrs. Stone sat down with the pediatrician. She tried to explain how she felt. Something was wrong with Christopher. Sometimes Chris seems to ignore all the sounds around him. When someone knocks on the door or the telephone rings, Chris doesn't turn around. "Is there something wrong with his hearing?" questioned Mrs. Stone.

Dr. Ross tried to reassure Mrs. Stone. "Chris really seems fine. He has been eating and growing. He hasn't had any serious diseases or infections. No one in your family is deaf. You didn't have German measles while you were pregnant. Why don't you wait a little while longer, and then we'll take a closer look if it still seems to be a concern."

The Stones waited, like so many parents do, until Christopher was twenty months old. By then, most children are beginning to talk and some are beginning to put words together. Chris seemed to understand a few words, but he didn't talk at all. "We must do something right now," Mrs. Stone declared. "I know that it's very important to detect a hearing loss while a child is young."

## DIAGNOSIS OF A HEARING LOSS

The signs and symptoms that Mrs. Stone noted in Christopher's case are some of the first observations that a specially

[2

trained doctor, or speech and hearing specialist, might make. In addition, children with a hearing loss will often laugh less than normal, hearing children. They may also bang their heads or stamp their feet just to feel the vibrations. Children with a hearing loss may also have a lot of temper tantrums to call attention to themselves or to show their feelings.

It's difficult to test for a hearing loss in newborn babies, but new tests are being developed. Speech and hearing clinics in hospitals are often better able to test for a hearing loss than the local family doctor. Tests usually involve recording how a baby acts when it hears a sudden loud noise. Some tests use film to record how the baby acts. Newer tests are more complicated. When a baby hears a sudden loud noise, it might breath faster. Its heart might beat faster. These changes are recorded on special machines. Even electrical changes that happen in the baby's brain can be recorded on a special machine called an *electroencephalograph.* If the child is older, a specially trained person called an *audiologist* may use a machine called an *audiometer* to find out if there is a hearing loss and to determine how bad the loss might be.

## CAUSES OF A
## HEARING LOSS

Because of health problems before or shortly after they are born, some babies are called high risk infants. They are more likely than other children to be born with a hearing loss, or to develop a hearing loss after birth. These children are watched very closely and tested more often than other children. A baby whose mother had *rubella* (German measles) when she first became pregnant would be at risk. If another person in the family was born deaf, the baby would also be a high risk.

[3

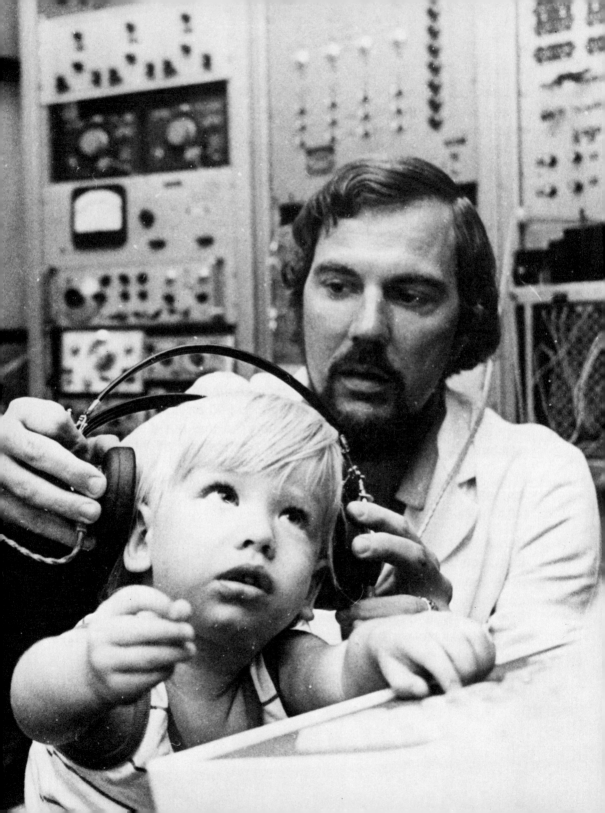

A baby born prematurely or a baby with another birth defect, such as brain damage, might also have a hearing loss. If a baby had many high fevers or serious ear infections or took certain drugs, it might also develop a hearing loss.

According to the *Annual Survey of Hearing Impaired Children and Youth in the United States,* the three greatest causes of hearing loss before a baby is born (prenatal causes) are: maternal rubella (its mother having had German measles while pregnant); heredity (deafness in the family); and complications due to prematurity (being born before nine months). The same survey explains that the three greatest causes of a hearing loss after a baby is born (postnatal causes) are: meningitis (an infection of the covering around the brain); measles; and otitis media (fluid in the middle ear). Sometimes, however, we don't know how or aren't able to pinpoint the reason for a child's hearing loss.

According to the U.S. Department of Health, Education and Welfare, the number of children in the United States who have a significant hearing handicap is about one million, although not all of these children were born with the hearing loss. Approximately 12 out of every 10,000 children are totally deaf and 150 to 300 out of every 10,000 children have a serious hearing loss.

*With the aid of a young "laboratory assistant," Dr. William Yost of the University of Florida is developing methods to diagnose hearing problems in the very young.*

Some experts feel that the number of young children who are either deaf or who have a severe hearing loss is increasing in the United States. It seems that medical progress has found ways to help most high risk unborn and newborn children to live, but with a hearing loss. Experts feel, however, that there are ways to lower the number of babies born with a hearing loss. Preventing injuries at birth and preventing prematurity should help. It is important, too, that babies that are particularly small when born receive special care. Also, if pregnant women do not take certain drugs or get certain diseases, such as German measles, fewer babies may be born with a hearing loss.

## WHO ARE THE HEARING-IMPAIRED?

According to most authorities, the term "hearing-impaired" includes all children who have a hearing impairment serious enough to warrant some type of special education services. The term involves both the labels "deaf" and "hard-of-hearing," which are classifications based essentially on the degree of hearing loss.

# Chapter 2
# HOW WE HEAR–
# OR DON'T HEAR

Think for a moment about how you hear. You may know that you use your ears and your brain to help you hear and understand what you have heard. To have a clear picture about how you are able to hear, you need to know some important facts about your ears; what they look like and how they work.

## ANATOMY OF THE EAR

The ear is made up of three parts; the *outer ear,* the *middle ear,* and the *inner ear.* The *pinna* is the part of the outer ear that you can see. Its job is to collect sounds and funnel them into the *external ear canal.* This canal is a short tunnel in the outer ear which leads to the *eardrum.* When sound waves hit the eardrum, also called the *tympanic membrane,* it begins to vibrate.

Past the eardrum lies the middle ear. Three bones, called *ossicles,* are in the air-filled space beyond the eardrum. The three bones are called *malleus* (hammer), *incus* (anvil), and *stapes* (stirrup) largely because they look somewhat like a hammer, an anvil, and a stirrup. These bones work like levers to move the sound waves from the eardrum to the inner ear. The *Eustachian tube* is also found in the middle ear. Its job is to help keep the right amount of air in the middle ear.

The inner ear is filled with fluid. It is here that the *end organs* for balance and hearing are located. The end organ for hearing is called the *cochlea.* It looks like a snail shell lined with little hairs. The cochlea is separated from the middle ear by two thin coverings called the *oval* and *round windows.* When the third bone in the middle ear, the stirrup, hits the oval window, the fluid in the inner ear begins to move, or vibrate. This movement of the fluid makes some of the cells in the cochlea give off a chemical electrical message called an *impulse.* The message then moves along the *auditory nerve* until it reaches the brain.

There is a special part of the brain called the *temporal lobes* which receive most of the messages connected with hearing. It is in the brain that we understand and interpret what has been heard.

*The Outer Ear. The auricle (pinna) funnels sound waves into the ear canal. The sound waves then cause the eardrum to vibrate.*

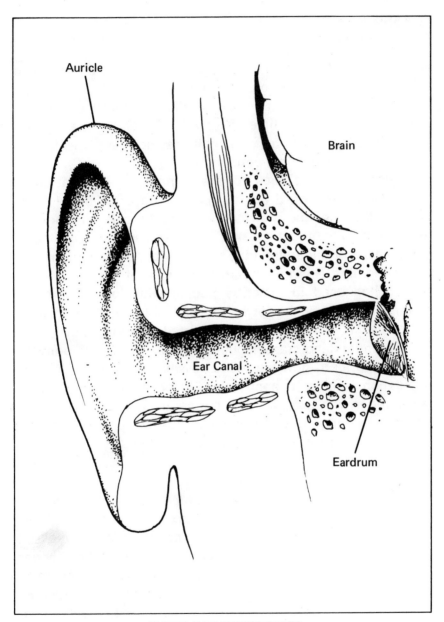

**OUTER EAR STRUCTURES**

## CLASSIFICATION
## OF HEARING LOSS

Have you ever had a bad head cold with a stuffed up nose and blocked ears? Maybe you have had a serious ear infection, and fluid has built up in your ears, making it difficult for you to hear properly. Sometimes people have a slight hearing loss for a short period of time. Sometimes, however, the loss is greater and may become permanent.

Loss of hearing does not mean the same thing as deafness. Usually the word deaf is used to describe people who have so little hearing that they are unable to learn language from listening to others speak. They often have difficulty learning to speak or understand the spoken word even with the use of hearing aids. Hearing-impaired and hard-of-hearing are two terms often used to describe people with some degree of hearing loss. They, however, are still able to learn at least some speech, sometimes with the use of a hearing aid.

To understand classifications of hearing loss, it is important first to learn how we measure what the normal hearing population is able to hear. Intensity of sound (loudness) is measured in *decibels* (db). The normal hearing population has an intensity range of 0–20 decibels (db) for speech. The best sensitivity for hearing is known as the *threshold.* The level

*The Middle Ear. The vibration of the eardrum activates three bones called the malleus, incus, and stapes. These bones in turn conduct the movement of sound waves from the eardrum to the inner ear.*

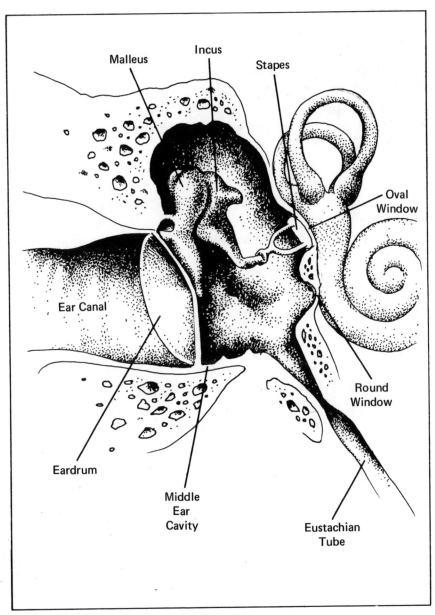

Malleus

Incus

Stapes

Oval
Window

Ear Canal

Round
Window

Eardrum

Middle
Ear
Cavity

Eustachian
Tube

**MIDDLE EAR STRUCTURES**

(db) at which a person is able to just detect a certain tone is called the threshold for that tone, or frequency.

A mild hearing loss is usually considered to be a loss ranging between 21 db and 40 db. A person with a mild hearing loss would have difficulty hearing faint or distant speech. In addition, that same person's own speech would seem almost normal, with perhaps only minor distortions or omissions of some sounds.

A moderate hearing loss is usually a loss in the range between 41 db and 55 db. If the loss is in both ears (a *bilateral loss*), the person will often find it hard to follow conversations of normal loudness at a distance of more than 3 to 6 feet (.9 to 1.8 m) from the speakers. This person's speech will usually have many errors in pronunciation, especially with consonant sounds such as Sue and shoe.

A moderately severe loss is usually a loss ranging between 56 db and 70 db. A person with this type of loss would be unable to follow a conversation unless the speakers spoke loudly and were standing very close to the person with the hearing loss. It would be difficult for a person with a moderately severe loss to function in a group. In addition, this person would probably have limited vocabulary and language skills. His or her speech would often be poor, with many errors in pronunciation and might have a hollow sound to it. A hearing aid will often help a person with this type of loss.

A severe hearing loss lies between 71 db and 90 db. If a person has this type of loss with both ears (bilateral loss), then it will be most difficult for him or her to follow a conversation. He or she may hear single words at a distance of about one foot (30 cm) and may be able to hear some loud sounds nearby. Even with hearing aids, however, this person still won't be able to hear speech clearly. It will be difficult for him or her to follow even simple sentences without vis-

[12

ual aids. A person with a severe hearing loss will require specialized help to produce understandable speech, but even then, this person's speech will most likely be very difficult to understand and will have an abnormal voice quality. This is especially true if a person becomes deaf before he or she has learned any language.

A profound hearing loss is often said to exist when the threshold lies above 90 db. If it is a bilateral loss, then most likely the person will react only once in a while to a very loud sound. A person with a profound hearing loss cannot rely on hearing for communication, even with the help of hearing aids. This person's speech usually can't be understood, although with special training, the person may be able to produce some words that other people can recognize. Again, this is particularly true if the person becomes deaf before he or she learned to speak. A person with this type of loss often uses *manual language* (sign language) or *total communication* (sign language while talking).

## TYPES OF HEARING LOSS

A *conductive hearing loss* is usually temporary and requires some medical treatment. It is generally caused by upper respiratory infections, fluid in the middle ear, too much wax in the ear, foreign objects in the auditory canal, or an abnormality in the structure of the external ear canal or middle ear.

A *sensorineural hearing loss* is caused by damage to the sensory cells in the cochlea, or nerve pathway leading to the brain. A loss of this type is almost always permanent and may become worse over time. The use of hearing aids to help a person with a sensorineural hearing loss to hear better is often recommended. Some of the causes of a sensorineural

[13

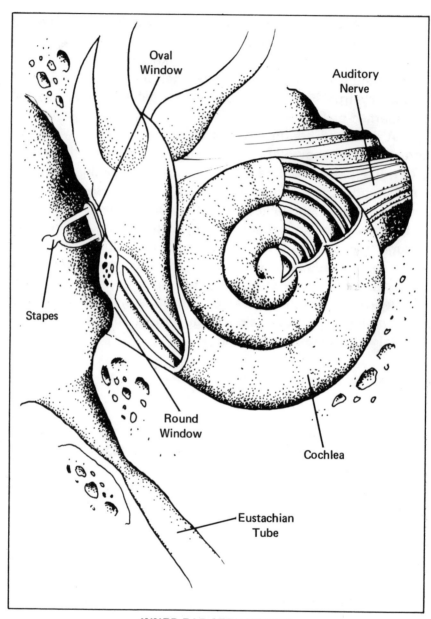

**INNER EAR STRUCTURES**

hearing loss include the mother contracting German measles during the first three months of pregnancy, a serious illness accompanied by very high fevers, the taking of certain drugs which damage the auditory nerve, a serious injury, being deprived of oxygen at birth or thereafter, and a problem with blood incompatibility (RH factor) between the pregnant mother and the baby before it is born. A mixed hearing loss is a sensorineural impairment combined with a conductive problem.

A *psychogenic hearing loss* is caused by emotional problems. A very frightening event or other major disturbance in a person's life may cause him or her to develop a hearing problem, when there is actually no physical reason for the hearing loss.

A *central auditory problem* is rather rare. The incoming sound is able to be heard but the person is not able to attach any meaning to that sound. A central auditory problem could be caused by a breakdown in the brain. Most children with this type of loss have been labeled in categories ranging from autistic to severely retarded. They usually have many other problems, besides central auditory dysfunction.

## MEDICAL TREATMENT

Sometimes a person must have surgery to correct or help the condition causing the hearing loss. For example, if a tumor was causing the problem, surgery might be required to re-

*The Inner Ear. The movement in the middle ear creates vibrations in the cochlea, where they are transformed into electrical energy and are carried to the brain.*

[15

move the tumor. At other times, medication is given to the person with a hearing loss. This is usually the case for conditions like ear infections involving a buildup of fluid in the ears, causing a temporary hearing loss. The doctor might give the person an antibiotic to clear up the infection, and some other medication to dry up the fluid.

Hearing aids are most often used to help people who have a hearing loss. These aids transmit sounds electronically and make them louder. A device called an ear mold is placed right into the person's external ear. This way, sounds are brought close to the inner ear and the auditory nerve. The amplifier which is used to make the sounds louder may be carried in a number of places. It may be put in a shirt or coat pocket or worn on the body as part of a harness. The amplifier may be built into the sides of eyeglasses or fitted onto the outer portion (pinna) of the ear. Although the most common fitting used to be monaural (one ear), there have recently been more people using aids for both ears (a binaural fitting).

It is wrong to think that a hearing aid will allow a person to hear perfectly. Hearing aids by themselves rarely improve a person's ability to make fine discriminations of speech sounds. Sometimes, in fact, the aid distorts or changes sounds. They may make it more difficult to hear small differences between sounds, especially sounds in words.

When deciding which type of hearing aid to use, several things are taken into consideration. The first important fact to consider is which hearing aid will improve the person's hearing with the least reduction in speech discrimination. The person who is going to use the aid might have a preference for where the amplifier will be kept. In addition, the cost of the hearing aid and the availability of service facilities to care for and monitor the hearing aid's use are also important details to consider when purchasing one.

[16

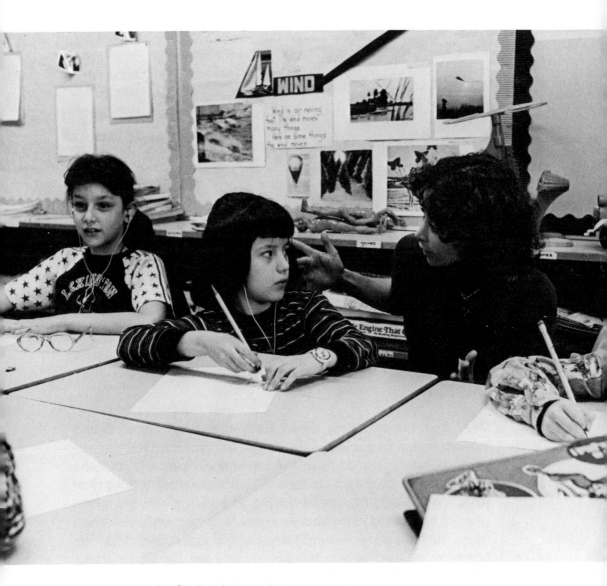

*At the Lexington School for the Deaf,
in New York City, hearing aids help these
children hear their teacher's instructions.*

# Chapter 3
# THE HEARING-IMPAIRED CHILD

"Deaf and dumb." How often Sara has been taunted and teased with those cruel words. She was born with a serious hearing loss and does have trouble speaking clearly, but she is definitely *not* stupid. Indeed, when nonverbal intelligence tests that do not require the child to hear or talk are given to deaf or hearing-impaired youngsters, it has generally been found that they are not inferior in intelligence. But Sara has had to work very hard to be accepted by her family, teachers, and friends. Most important, she has had to learn to feel good about herself.

## THE EFFECTS OF DEAFNESS
## ON THE INDIVIDUAL

When Sara was very young, she, like other normal children, had to depend a great deal on other people. However, Sara's deafness made her depend on others for a longer period of time than most other children. For this reason, deaf or hearing-impaired children are often considered somewhat more immature than normal children. When Sara was young, her parents did too many things for her that she was fully capable of doing for herself. Her brothers and sisters all helped her clean her room, get dressed, make snacks, and do household chores. What Sara really needed was for her family to make more demands on her.

Often deaf children with deaf parents will mature more easily and quickly than deaf children with hearing parents. The deaf children can usually communicate more easily with their deaf parents by using manual means of communication, such as body and sign language. This is usually easier for a deaf parent. Deaf parents will also tend to place more demands on their deaf children and thus help them become independent sooner.

Hearing-impaired youngsters do, however, tend to have more behavioral problems than their hearing counterparts. Hearing-impaired children may be more quiet than other children. They may keep more to themselves, and give in to others, more often than normal children.

When Sara was very young, she had what some considered to be an inferiority complex. She didn't have much confidence in herself. She would often be very quiet and spend a great deal of time by herself. But when she entered high

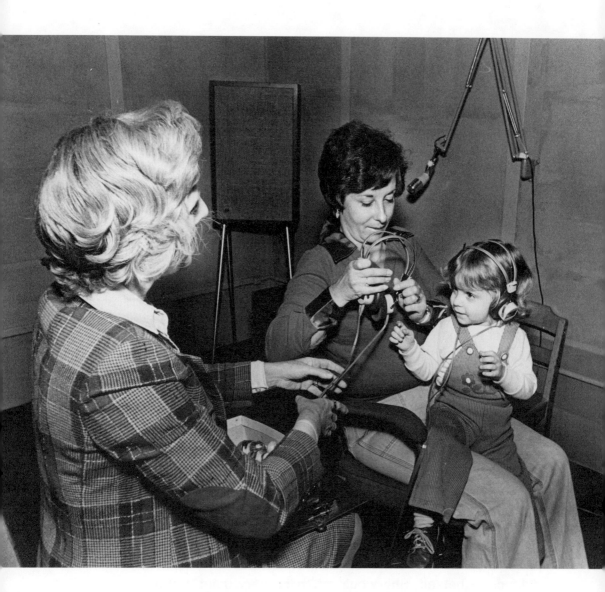

*Special audiological tests are helpful in diagnosing hearing problems in young children.*

school, she came out of her shell, matured a great deal, and seemed happy and well-adjusted.

A man named Hans Furth has spent many years studying deafness. He has found that when most hearing-impaired children reach adolescence and adulthood, they often become well-adjusted. Indeed, Furth feels that a deaf adolescent does not go through many of the problems a hearing adolescent faces. Furth believes that deaf youngsters actually live in a simpler world than their hearing counterparts. Because of this simplicity, the most important crisis of a deaf child's adjustment appears to be the conscious acceptance of his or her deafness and the limitations this handicap presents. This acceptance is, according to Furth, very important to the deaf child's long-term well-being. He feels that a typical deaf adult is an extrovert who is highly dependent on sign language for communication. A deaf adult has only a few close relationships with hearing persons. Most of the deaf adult's fulfillment comes from finding companionship, friendship, love, marriage, amusement, sports, and religion within the deaf community.

Several surveys have been done through the years looking at different aspects of the lives of deaf adults. How they feel about themselves, their relationships to family and friends, and their employment records are included in the information gathered by these surveys. Most of the data concerning employment of deaf people revealed that the quality and reliability of deaf workers was consistently good. Unfortunately, some surveys found that the deaf face similar barriers to their acceptance for employment and training as some racial, religious, and social minorities do. Discrimination in job placement and advancement for the hearing-impaired does exist. However, with the new emphasis on mainstreaming in public schools—that is, integrating the hearing-impaired into the normal school population—it is hoped that the deaf will be viewed as persons with characteristics that may make them distinct, but no less equal than everyone else.

## THE EFFECTS OF DEAFNESS
## ON THE FAMILY

When Sara's parents first found out that Sara had a severe hearing problem, they were extremely upset. This time of real grief then changed to a period when her parents almost refused to believe that Sara had a serious hearing loss. They searched all over for the "right" doctor or the "right" cure. After this time of protesting, Sara's parents then went through periods of despair when they tried to separate themselves from Sara because it was so painful for them to accept having a child with a serious handicap. Finally, Sara's parents accepted the fact that she did have a severe hearing loss. Individual and group counseling, discussion groups, and general education about deafness for her parents, brothers, and sisters really helped her family to accept Sara's handicap.

Not all families have as much difficulty accepting a child with a hearing loss. How parents may feel depends on a number of things. Some parents whose children are diagnosed as severely deaf will accept the diagnosis more quickly than parents of hard-of-hearing children. If parents are told that their child is hard-of-hearing but there didn't seem to be any real medical cause, they may react with the greatest amount of disbelief. The kind of hearing loss, the degree of the loss, each family member's individual personality, the relationship of family members to one another, the ages of the brothers and sisters, and the overall stability of the family may all affect how well the hearing-impaired child is accepted.

The environment a family creates for the deaf child is very important. First, the family needs to capitalize on any hearing the child may have. Careful attention should be given to make sure the child's hearing aid is working and is kept in good repair. It is also important to be sure that wax does not build up in the child's ears. The family needs to work as a team to constantly increase the deaf child's vocabulary and encourage the child to use language as much as possible. The family should work cooperatively in speech and language training. Learning sign language may be a way to help family members communicate better.

There are many ways in which the family can help the deaf youngster become an integral part of the family. First of all, the hearing-impaired child should be included in family activities such as outings, trips, and projects. Family members can talk and sing with the deaf child, take the youngster shopping and visiting, and introduce him or her to new places and experiences. The deaf child should also be included in family work activities. This will help the child learn to be self-sufficient, self-reliant, independent, and sociable.

## THE EFFECT OF DEAFNESS ON PEER RELATIONS

Sara had trouble making friends when she went to school. Because many of the children there did not understand about deafness, they were afraid of Sara and made fun of her. Children all too often take out their frustrations on a handicapped child.

The federal government recently passed a new special education law, which tries to encourage all youngsters with special needs to be mainstreamed into regular classrooms to the greatest extent possible. Many youngsters with a wide variety of special needs are coming into classrooms with normal children for the first time. Because this is a big change for many parents, teachers, and students, everyone must work together to make this new program effective.

At the preschool level, children usually tend to accept a deaf child easily. It is not really necessary to bring up the subject of the hearing aid until someone notices it and asks questions. It may be days or weeks before the other children notice the aid, unless it is worn conspicuously. The easiest way to explain the aid is the most direct way: "Some of us don't see well. Our eyes don't work the way they should, so we have to wear glasses. Sara's ears don't work the way they should, so she has to wear a hearing aid. It makes everything louder so Sara can hear better." The children should be told not to bump into the child's ears. They should also be told not to shout. They need to talk noticeably, but close, so that they can be heard more clearly.

One of the goals of mainstreaming special needs students into regular classrooms is to improve attitudes of people toward special needs youngsters. One study tried to look at how successfully deaf and hearing-impaired students were being mainstreamed. The study found that hearing-impaired children with very few language skills formed their own special group. They excluded children with normal hearing and other hearing-impaired children. Hearing-impaired children who had the best verbal language skills seemed to interact much more frequently with their normal hearing peers. The

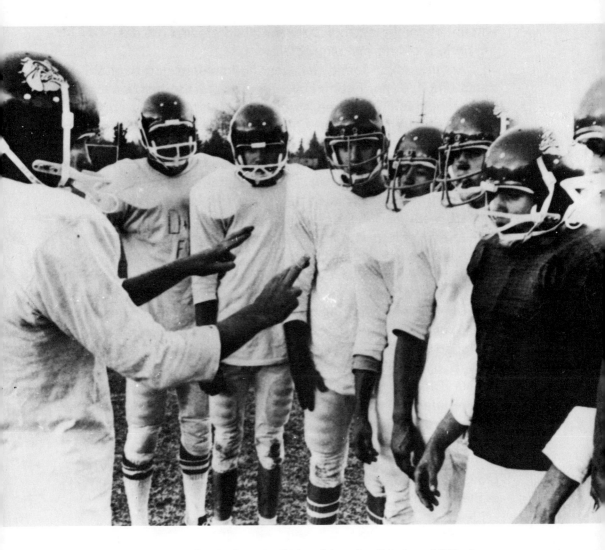

Members of the Colorado School for the Deaf and Blind
football team watch their quarterback as he
uses sign language to call a play.

amount of communication between children was greatest during periods of informal play activity.

Another study found that hearing-impaired and deaf students directed more communication toward the teacher than other students. This same study also found that the normal hearing children talked and played more with more children than did the hearing-impaired children.

Although the studies do point out some of the limitations of the mainstreaming efforts, hearing-impaired youngsters are becoming more of an integral part of the entire community. Indeed, deaf and hearing-impaired people are being welcomed more often into society. Special sign language translators have been added to important programs on television. The news captioned for the deaf can usually be seen on television each day. Increased captioning of regular TV broadcasts began on major American networks in January, 1980. These captions can only be seen if the television set is equipped with a special decoder. "Sesame Street," a widely viewed children's television program, has had many deaf guests come on the program to visit and share some of their unique talents. Television specials have been aired on major networks depicting stories of deaf children and deaf adults. Special sign language courses are now being offered at colleges and universities across the United States. Many religious groups throughout the country are using sign language at their services.

# Chapter 4
# THE LEARNING PROCESS

"If that teacher says it to me one more time, I think I'll scream! I know I'm not stupid. My math is great, sure. But those word problems are going to kill me. What does he want me to do?" sighed Steve.

Bill tried to help his good friend. "Look, Mr. Cronin really cares. He knows word problems are tough, but he wants to help. Steve, you're just about the fastest calculator in the class. There must be something we can do to pull up your average. With a few more points you'll be okay, and you'll be able to play at Saturday's basketball game. Sit down with Cronin after school. Work it out."

# THE EFFECTS OF DEAFNESS
## ON ACADEMIC SKILLS

Steve has a hearing impairment. He, like other hard-of-hearing and deaf students, typically has trouble with school subjects that rely most heavily on verbal skills. A study done by Gallaudet College found that hearing-impaired students do better in reading than in other academic areas during the first one to three years of education, but thereafter, achieve higher grades in mathematics and lower grades in verbal subjects.

This same study also found that there was a relationship between the degree of hearing loss and achievement. The more severe the hearing loss, the poorer the student performed in the area of reading comprehension. Students with the greatest hearing loss perform better in low-verbal and nonverbal academic areas, such as spelling and arithmetic computation.

It takes about three years to prepare typical deaf children for the first grade. It usually takes between ten to twelve years for deaf children to complete the elementary grades. Deaf students are usually two or more years behind normal students in educational achievement. The average deaf pupil who earns a high school diploma—often at nineteen or twenty years of age—is about two years behind the average high school graduate in overall academic achievement. Some students can graduate from college. Indeed, Gallaudet College in Washington, D.C., is designed for deaf students. Some hearing-impaired students do go to regular colleges, graduate, and compete successfully in the hearing world. Indeed, some even go on to get masters and doctoral degrees.

# THE EFFECTS OF DEAFNESS
## ON INTELLIGENCE

"Steve, I'm not trying to pick on you. I've looked through your records and spoken with the guidance counselor. You're a bright kid. You calculate perfectly and do it faster than anyone else in the class. With your intelligence, I know you can do better with these word problems," stated Mr. Cronin.

"Mr. Cronin," replied Steve, "do me a favor and speak to Ms. Miller. She works with me a lot, you know, kind of like a tutor. Maybe she's got some ideas or can figure something out."

The Ms. Miller Steve was referring to was his resource room teacher. Ms. Miller is a specially trained teacher who is used to working with hearing-impaired students. When Mr. Cronin stopped in, she was expecting him.

"Steve told me you might drop by. He's really upset about his math average—something about not playing in Saturday's game. Word problems are really hard for him. What can I do to help?" questioned Ms. Miller.

"I don't think Steve's trying. The rest of his work in math is great," answered Mr. Cronin. "Besides, I know he's really smart. Why isn't he doing better?"

"Steve has had a hearing impairment for many years," Ms. Miller began. "He is bright, as are many deaf kids, and he was lucky to have been given educational opportunities at a very early age to help him develop to his fullest potential. But subjects that require a lot of language, something like word problems in math, are very difficult for even bright deaf children. I'll try to give him extra help after school for a while. In the meantime, please believe that Steve is trying, and in

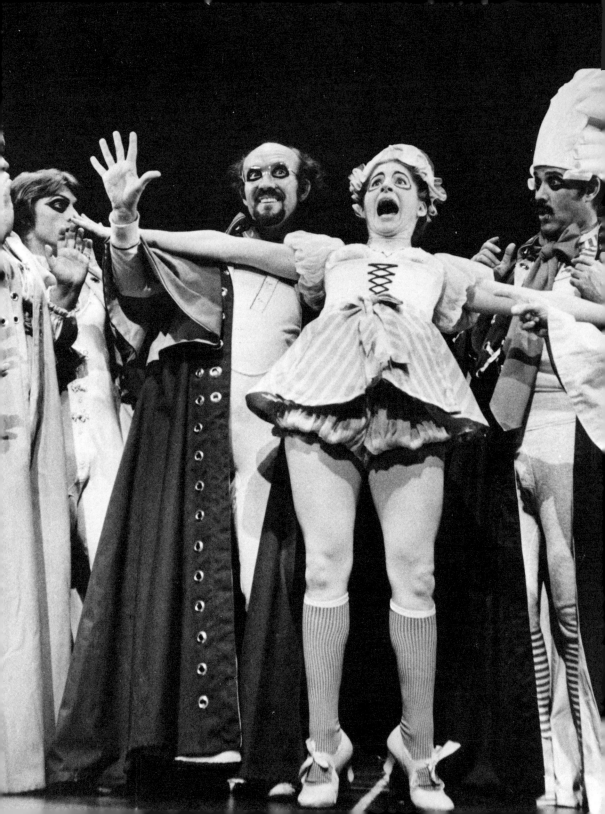

time, he'll improve. Saturday's game is very important to him. If he could play, I know it would mean a great deal to him."

Before Mr. Cronin spoke with Ms. Miller, he really believed that Steve was not trying very hard to do the word problems correctly. He kept thinking that because Steve was smart, he should do better. In one sense, that is a positive happening. Most people don't realize that deaf and hearing-impaired people are intelligent. Too often the phrase "deaf and dumb" has been used to describe people who are hard-of-hearing.

Intelligence has been studied, measured, and defined by many different authorities. Piaget, a famous Swiss psychologist, outlined several stages that make up a child's intellectual growth and development. According to Piaget's theory, a child is able to differentiate him or herself from others at approximately one and one-half to two years of age. The deaf child, Furth feels, is also able to distinguish between him or herself and others at this age. Symbol formation—the ability to attach an abstract symbol to a meaningful object—usually occurs next in a child's intellectual growth and development. For example, a young child of about two years of age will connect the word 'ball' with an actual ball. A hearing child usually will begin to use verbal language or "conventional symbols" at this stage of development. The deaf child, according to Furth, will begin to depend on "motivated sym-

*Most, but not all of the actors in the National Theatre of the Deaf, are actually deaf themselves. They play to both hearing and deaf audiences all around the country.*

[31

bols" such as play and gestures. These "motivated symbols" are produced out of a sense of need—that is, the deaf child's need to communicate in some fashion.

Although much learning does occur through the use of verbal skills, language alone does not provide all knowledge. Indeed, from a developmental point of view, play and gestures are initially more important to a child's intellectual development. A typical five-year-old deaf child has intelligence, is able to organize the world around him or herself, has symbolic skills such as play and gestures, and has some communicative skills. The deaf child, however, does not have a linguistic system.

It has been reported that there is a slight lag in intellectual functioning of a deaf child around the time of middle childhood, usually between six and ten years of age. The intellectual development of children goes from what has been defined by Piaget as concrete thinking to formal thinking. It is this shift from concrete to more abstract thought that is most difficult for the deaf child. Failure to master a verbal language will not prevent a person from achieving the level of formal thought. However, Furth feels that lack of motivation, or desire to do so, will. At this stage of intellectual development it becomes very important for the deaf to *want* to continue to learn if he or she is to reach full intellectual potential.

Mental development of the deaf is reported to be related to the deaf child's environment. It seems to be very important to provide hearing-impaired youngsters with surroundings rich in learning situations and language. Specialists point out that there are some very important or critical periods during which intellectual development needs to take place. If a child waits to learn until he or she enters school, that youngster may be very frustrated. Being unable to communicate with family members builds up huge frustrations in children and may lower a child's eventual intellectual level. The preschool years when the brain is growing so fast, and the youngster has a tremendous natural drive to learn are seen as the most important time to begin learning.

To measure intellectual ability, a trained psychologist usually administers an intelligence test. Early intelligence testing of the deaf population (beginning in the early 1900s) produced scores which placed many deaf people in the lower range of intelligence. It is very important to realize that most of the test instruments used at that time were meant to test hearing people, and generally relied heavily on language skills. Today, special tests are used to measure the intelligence of deaf people. These tests do not rely on language to any great extent. In addition, the people who give the test usually have had a great deal of practice working with deaf and hearing-impaired youngsters. When the appropriate tests are given by an experienced examiner, the intelligence of hearing-impaired people is generally no lower than that of the hearing population.

## THE EFFECTS OF DEAFNESS ON LEARNING VERBAL LANGUAGE

"Deaf and dumb" is a phrase which was heard more frequently in the past than today. Besides poor test results, deaf people had difficulty speaking and otherwise communicating with other people. The main reason for all this misunderstanding deals with the great difficulty hearing-impaired people have in learning verbal language. Think for a moment how important language is to you at home, with friends, and in school.

[33

In the normal hearing population, a young child first learns to understand oral language that is spoken to him or her. Next, the child will learn to express himself or herself by talking. Recognizable words are spoken at about one year of age. The deaf or hearing-impaired infant will cry and babble in much the same way a normal infant would. But before the child is one year old, however, it usually becomes noticeable that the child is not imitating sounds made by others.

The age at which the hearing loss occurs affects how easily the hearing-impaired child will acquire language. If the loss occurs from birth to eighteen months of age, it becomes very difficult to learn to speak. If the loss occurs after the child has already started talking, it is usually easier for oral language to develop.

How well a deaf person's speech is understood is somewhat related to the degree of the hearing loss; however, other factors can also affect the quality of speech. How smart the hearing-impaired person is, the type and quality of education received, and the desire to speak understandably are other things which affect how well a hearing-impaired person is understood.

There are some language skills which are more difficult for deaf students to master. Typically, idiomatic expressions, ("it's raining cats and dogs"), are very difficult to learn. Words with multiple meanings, such as bark (bark of a dog or bark of a tree), present difficulty in learning. Recent studies found that a slight hearing impairment usually reduces the amount of words as well as the types of words (such as nouns and verbs) that a youngster is able to learn. A moderate impairment lowers the use of adverbs, pronouns, and auxiliaries. A profound impairment reduces nearly all types of words.

# METHODS OF LEARNING SPEECH
# AND LANGUAGE IN THE DEAF
# OR HEARING-IMPAIRED CHILD

Steve attends classes with normal hearing students. He does receive some extra help with Ms. Miller, but for the most part, his education takes place in the mainstream of a public high school. Someone is present in each class to translate what the teacher says into sign language. Steve's parents feel that one of the major reasons he is able to do so well is because of the method that was used to teach him speech and language.

There are basically four methods for teaching deaf and hearing-impaired youngsters in use today. In the *oral method,* the student takes in information through a combination of lip reading and the use of a hearing aid. The hearing-impaired child expresses himself or herself through speech. In the *auditory method,* the student is taught to concentrate on developing listening skills. Reading, writing, and lipreading are discouraged. The auditory method is used primarily with children with moderate loss and sometimes with profoundly impaired youngsters. The *Rochester method* is a combination of the oral method with fingerspelling, which will be explained later on in this book. In the Rochester method, the student takes in information through lipreading, the use of a hearing aid, and fingerspelling. The student expresses himself or herself through speech and fingerspelling. Emphasis is placed on reading and writing. The *simultaneous method* is a combination of the oral method, sign language and fingerspelling. The student takes in information through lipreading, the use of a hearing aid, sign language, and fingerspelling. The youngster expresses himself

[35

or herself through speech, signs and fingerspelling. Sign language is a system of gestures using the hands and arms to suggest a particular thought. Fingerspelling is a method of forming the letters from A to Z with the fingers. The teacher using this method uses sign language as well as the spoken word.

Another method, known as *total communication,* is sometimes placed in the category of simultaneous communication. It has become quite popular in recent years and is now supported by the National Association of the Deaf. This method encourages the use of all forms of communication, including pantomime, fingerspelling, and sign language. According to some experts, the simultaneous use of signing and speaking is the most natural way to be understood.

Steve's parents had a great deal of difficulty finding a school which would utilize a teaching method they felt would be best for their son. Some schools use a purely oral approach to teaching speech and language. Indeed, the oral method has been the major method used in schools for the deaf for many years. The oral method relies heavily on lip-reading, a skill difficult to learn and tiring to use. Even when the listener is very close to the speaker, many sounds are easily confused. Advocates of this method feel that since we live in a "hearing world," the oral method allows the deaf child to become a part of our society more easily.

*At the 1979 Academy Awards, actress Jane Fonda used sign language as she accepted her Oscar for Best Performance by an Actress in a Leading Role, for her part in* Coming Home.

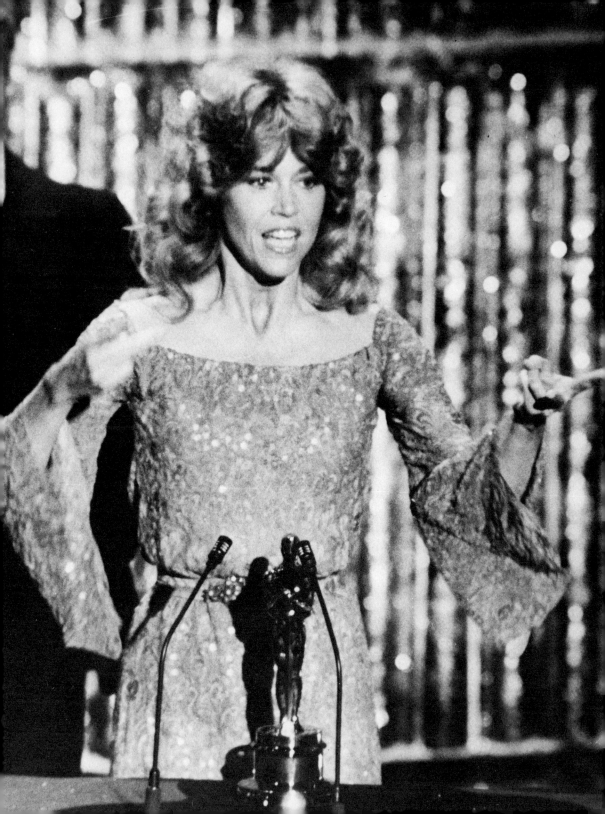

Manual communication, that is, the use of fingerspelling, sign language or gestures, despite some strong opposition from the hearing community, has survived. The critics of this form of communication argue that by using manual methods, the deaf child will be able to have social contacts only with those people who understand manual communication. In addition, they state that once the child has learned a manual method, he or she will be less motivated to try to learn the more difficult tasks of speech and lipreading. Advocates of manual means of communication argue that deaf children need some method of communication and will often learn manual communication informally from other children.

A major component of manual communication is American Sign Language, (A.S.L.). It has many forms. The most formal system is the manual alphabet, or fingerspelling. Most hearing-impaired people use both signs and fingerspelling in their conversations. Fingerspelling is used to spell out those words for which there are no signs. Usually, the more informal the setting, the more signs are used.

The major systems of American Sign Language are Native Sign Language, or Ameslan; and Signed English, or Senglish. Native Sign Language is the standard form of A.S.L. It uses a minimum of spelling, word order may not be the same as in English, and facial expressions and body postures are also used to convey meaning. Signed English is more formal than Native Sign Language. It uses most aspects of English, including word order. Signs and fingerspelling are used for this purpose.

Other systems of American Sign Language have been developed more recently. Seeing Essential English ($SEE_1$) was developed in 1962. This system has the largest vocabulary of any other system. Signing Exact English ($SEE_2$) was developed in 1972. Several other variations have been developed in recent years.

Steve's parents spoke to many experts and visited many schools before they were able to find one which utilized the total communications approach. In the past, schools only allowed total communication as a last resort. If it could be proven that a child could not learn at a reasonable rate using the oral method, usually by twelve years of age, then manual communication was sometimes introduced.

Because the method of total communication has spread so quickly, there is little standardization in its use; however, there have been excellent results reported. Furth has done a comparison of the progress made by two groups of students over a period of four years. One group was taught with the oral method and the other was taught with the Total Communication Approach. Furth found that the total communication group performed better on a test for reading skills and a test for knowledge of grammar. In fact, research seems to indicate that manual communication, especially when used very early in life, encourages intellectual growth. It also reduces the amount of frustration the young deaf child often feels at his or her inability to communicate with family and friends. Finally, the studies also tend to indicate that oral skills are not made worse by manual communication.

# Chapter 5
# HELPING THE HEARING-IMPAIRED

What caused my child's hearing loss? Was it my fault? Can it be cured? Will my child learn to talk? If so, when and how well? Where do I go for help? Where will my child be able to go to school? Can my child go to college?

These are but a few of the questions parents often ask themselves and others when they find out their child has a hearing impairment. Of all the questions asked, perhaps some of the most important are those related to the type of education the hearing-impaired youngster will receive.

The problem of educating hearing-impaired children is filled with controversy. Disagreement among experts centers on several topics. Some experts feel that deaf youngsters need to be taught through the use of the oral communication method, while others argue in favor of manual or total communication methods. Some experts believe hearing-impaired youngsters should live in a residential (boarding) school, while others feel a day school is better. The importance of mainstreaming into public schools is also a topic about which experts cannot seem to agree.

## CHOOSING THE RIGHT SCHOOL

There is no easy way to decide which type of educational program is best for the hearing-impaired child. Programs for children with a hearing loss vary according to the individual needs of the child and the facilities that the local community has available. Alternatives usually found outside public school systems include special residential schools and special day schools. Within public schools there may be classes in a separate wing of a building, or special classes mixed in among other classes in a school building. Or, there may be resource class arrangements with students spending some time each day in a resource room with a specialist and other time in regular classes. Finally, there may be regular class placement with special education services brought to the hearing-impaired youngsters by specialists who work with the classroom teachers and students right in the regular classroom.

Currently more than half of the deaf children in the United States are educated with their hearing counterparts in public schools. The number of deaf children in special boarding schools is declining.

It is most important to consider the requirements of a good educational program for the deaf when one is trying to decide where a hearing-impaired child should go to school.

[41

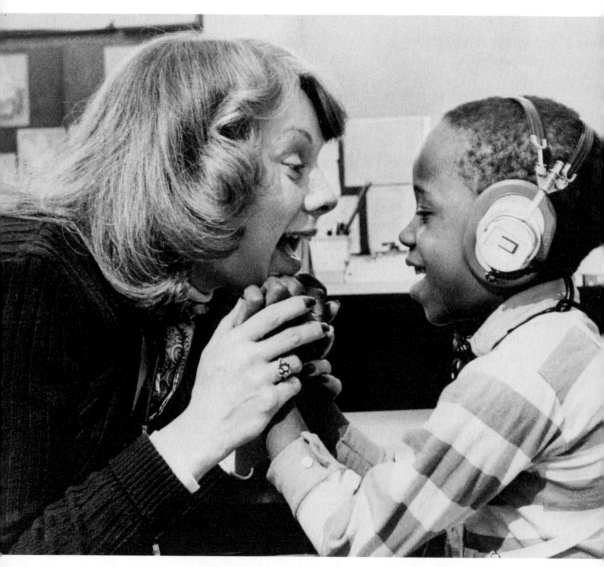

*This teacher is helping her student learn to
say a word by letting him feel her pronounce it.*

According to some authorities, a very important part of a good program is the teaching staff. Teachers should be trained to work with the deaf and they should be supervised by qualified people who are highly knowledgeable about the education of the deaf. Special help from people trained in psychology and audiology who are knowledgeable about deaf children and their problems should be available in a good educational setting. Opportunities for extracurricular activities such as sports, should also be available. Appropriate equipment such as amplification systems and captioned films should also be present in a school capable of teaching deaf students. Finally, some experts feel that there should also be provision for vocational training and counseling in a good school for hearing-impaired students.

## MAINSTREAMING
## HEARING-IMPAIRED STUDENTS

After the new federal special education law, Public Law 94–142, was passed, an increasing number of special needs students were being placed, to the greatest extent possible, in regular classrooms. There is a growing movement, not only in the United States, but also in England and Canada, to include hearing-impaired children in regular classrooms. Successful mainstreaming requires many different things. Among the most important issues to consider are the attitudes of parents, teachers, special needs students and regular education students toward mainstreaming efforts.

Many parents of normal children will be in favor of having children with special needs in the classroom. In some cases, however, parents do object. Prejudice is sometimes caused by a lack of understanding or information. A better understanding of the reasons for placing children with their normal peer groups can lead to better attitudes. A positive attitude by the classroom teacher can also help parents develop more positive attitudes themselves.

Attitudes of parents of the hearing-impaired children can be improved by encouraging parents to become involved in some way with the school. A classroom teacher may help the hearing-impaired child's parents get to know the school. An understanding of the school's program and the development of a good relationship with the whole staff often improves the parents' attitudes. Letting parents observe their child in school might also be helpful. Periodic conferences between parents and teachers and parent education programs are also useful in helping to develop positive attitudes toward the mainstreaming process.

Teachers themselves have certain concerns, especially a first-time teacher of a child with a hearing loss. If a child doesn't respond immediately, the teacher may wonder if the child has heard what was said. The teacher needs to know that the hearing-impaired youngster must not be overprotected. Normal student behavior needs to be encouraged. Any special services that the hearing-impaired child is receiving should be fully explained to the teacher. Knowledge about hearing and deafness will help the teacher feel more competent and at ease in dealing with special students.

Attitudes of both the hearing-impaired and normal hearing students about themselves and each other are critical to the mainstreaming process. It is important to remember that *every* student is a member of the class. The sense of belonging to that group will help each student learn better and feel better about him or herself.

When a hearing-impaired student is mainstreamed into a

[44

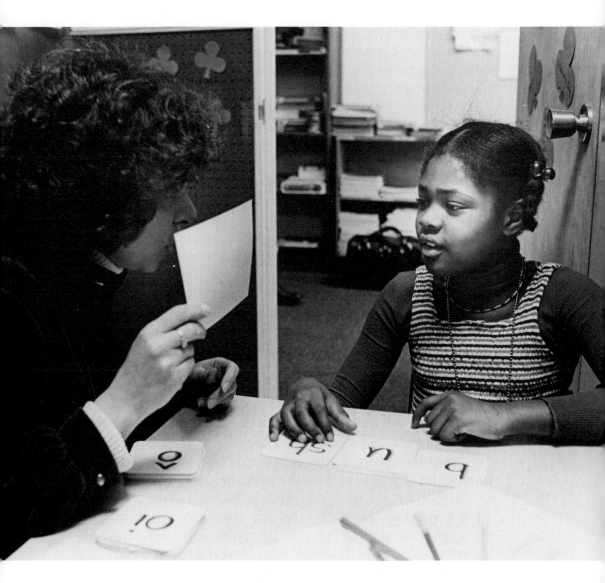

*One-to-one lessons in speech and auditory
training are helpful to deaf students.*

regular classroom, authorities suggest that the child sit in a location that will lessen the strain of listening and allow the best opportunity to lipread and watch facial expressions to aid in understanding. To begin with, the hearing-impaired child should sit as close to the teacher and as far away from distracting noise sources as possible. If a child has one better ear, then the child should be seated with the better ear toward the teacher and away from unnecessary noise. If both ears are the same, then sitting in the middle, rather than to one side, would be the better place. The hearing-impaired child should also be allowed to move around the class to hear better.

In many instances, a hearing-impaired child who is main-streamed into a regular classroom will also attend a resource room for part of the day. The purpose of this is usually to tutor the child according to his or her specific needs, including speech correction, lipreading instruction, auditory training, language instruction, and even academic subjects such as science, math, or social studies. Even the location of the re-source room is an important point to consider. It should be easy to reach by both students and teachers. It should be within the physical plant of the school and be located at a place which will enable classroom teachers and the resource teachers to talk together easily.

The curriculum, or subjects taught in the classroom, may have to be changed a little for hearing-impaired youngsters. One important thing to consider is that the hard-of-hearing child may be exhausted by the effort of remaining constantly alert for long periods of time. If possible, the hearing-im-paired student should have shorter lesson periods or perhaps be allowed to take a short rest period in between classes.

Very often, hearing-impaired youngsters may be excluded from class activities such as music or dancing, or social activities and functions. The hard-of-hearing child should be encouraged to participate in these activities. Music and dancing, for example, might very well help improve the child's rhythm and discrimination of sounds.

When audio-visual equipment is used in the classroom, it is very important that the hard-of-hearing child be able to see and hear the equipment adequately. If the child is to listen to a tape recorder, it would be useful to have some kind of picture or book to go with the recording. Listening to a tape recorder should be done in small groups, with earphones which can be individually adjusted.

When tests are given to the class, it is often a good idea to give the hearing-impaired child the test individually, or in a small group. This would allow the child to take the test at a slower speed. Some tests may not be right for a hearing-impaired child, and should not be used at all.

The choice of textbooks requires careful consideration. When possible, texts with complicated vocabulary and complex language structures should be avoided. It is a good idea to provide the hearing-impaired child with other options for learning besides a text. For example, a science experiment might provide the same learning experience as a chapter in a science text. There are some materials designed especially for use by deaf students, but these are most often used in resource rooms or self-contained classrooms rather than a regular classroom setting.

# Chapter 6
# OTHER WAYS
# TO COMMUNICATE

Have you ever thought how important it is to be able to hear? We rely on our hearing to learn and understand most of our language. Think how difficult it would be to communicate with family and friends if you couldn't listen to and understand much of what they said. What if your family and friends didn't understand you when you spoke? How would you feel?

Our sense of hearing allows us to follow events that might be out of our sight or reach. Hearing sometimes serves as a warning system. We sometimes hear something danger-ous before we can see it. Even when we are sleeping, our sense of hearing might help us wake up if there is danger. Hearing also can help create a background of mood or feeling. Did you ever listen to the music during a battle scene in a movie? Music helps to create a certain mood.

Although you might have perfect hearing, have you ever wondered how it might feel to have a hearing impairment? In this chapter there will be several suggested activities which might give you some idea of how it feels to have a hearing loss.

## LIPREADING

Lipreading is something hearing-impaired people often do to help them understand what is being said around them. In the oral method of communication, lipreading is critically important. But lipreading is not easy to do. It requires great concentration and is often very tiring. A hearing-impaired person must be able to see the speaker's mouth clearly if lipreading is to be done with success. Many words look alike when they are mouthed, which makes lipreading even more difficult. Often hearing-impaired people must use the meaning of the sentence to help them figure out what a particular word says.

You might want to try some lipreading with a friend. Have your friend mouth a short sentence and see if you can understand what is being said. Try to carry on a conversation by just mouthing your words. Is it easy for you to do? If you watched a television show without the sound, could you understand what was said? What if you had to do this most of the time?

There are some hints which can help you make lipreading easier. First of all, remember to watch the speaker's mouth. The speaker must not cover his or her mouth, or turn away. Also, the speaker needs to mouth the words as if he or she were speaking regularly, without overpronouncing the

[49

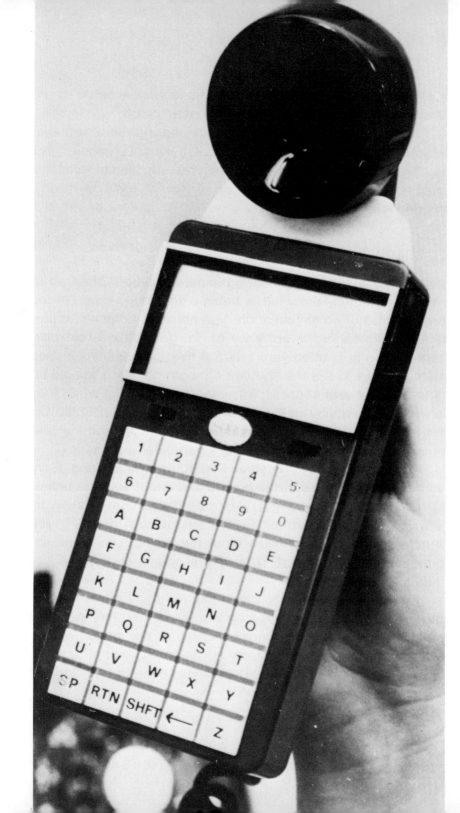

words. Exaggerated movements make it more difficult to understand. Long, complicated sentences should be avoided. The same information must be broken up into smaller parts.

## LEARNING TO TALK

Do you remember learning to talk? Most children begin saying words at about one year of age, and then begin putting words together to make short sentences by the time they're one and one half or two. Children usually imitate what they hear others say. Deaf children, however, really can't learn to talk by hearing others. They learn by watching other people very carefully. They watch the way people move their lips and jaws and tongues as they speak. Then, they try to copy what they see. In addition, deaf youngsters learn by feeling the vibrations that sounds make. They try to copy the same vibrations in their throats.

You may want to try to see how it feels to learn to talk when you are deaf. You will need the help of a friend. Place your fingers on your friend's throat to try to feel the vibrations as he or she speaks. Sometimes you can feel vibrations in the chest, nose, top of the head or back of the neck as well as on the throat. Notice the differences in vibrations between high and low sounds. Remember, a deaf person must also try to copy the same movements of the jaw, lips, and tongue of the speaker. You'll see that this is not very easy to do.

*Engineers have developed a portable device that allows deaf people to communicate better over the telephone.*

Here is an exercise which will give you an idea of how deaf people learn to speak. Have your partner think of a word, but not tell you what it is. Next, your partner should hum the sounds that would be made if the word was being said, *without* mouthing the word. Feel the vibrations of your partner's body and try to copy the humming. Next, have your partner hum the word and mouth it at the same time. Now you must copy the humming and the movements of your partner's lips, tongue and jaw. Can you guess what the word is?

## HEARING AIDS

If you have never seen a hearing aid, you might want to invite an audiologist to speak with your class in school. This person could bring several types of aids to your classroom, and explain how they work and how to take care of them.

If you have an opportunity to try on the aid, it might be interesting for you to hear how sounds are magnified. You'll probably learn that sounds are not necessarily made more clear, they are just made louder. Indeed, sometimes the amplification of the sounds will make speech less clear.

## MIME, SIGNALS
## AND BODY LANGUAGE

We use many ways to communicate other than speaking. Think about the times you nodded your head, shook your finger or fist at someone, smiled, or frowned. You were saying something to someone else without using words. Many people use gestures regularly as part of their jobs. Umpires in a baseball game use hand signals to call the plays. Conductors of orchestras use hand and body movements to signal members of the orchestras. Think about other workers you know who use signals as a regular part of their job. Try mime with a friend and see if your partner can understand what you are trying to say.

Body language can be a very powerful tool for conveying meaning, both for the deaf and for people with normal hearing. Often the deaf are more aware of their body movements and use them purposefully to convey meaning. Everyone uses body language, but most hearing people are unaware of all the meanings being conveyed through their bodies. Sometime you might want to videotape yourself in a normal conversation. When you view the tape, watch the way your body moves. What were you saying with your body? Did you mean to say all those things?

## SIGN LANGUAGE

Sign Language (often referred to simply as "sign") is used by many deaf and hearing-impaired people. Perhaps a deaf friend or a teacher of the deaf might be able to teach you some sign language. If you watch some special programs on television captioned for the hearing impaired, you might be able to learn some sign. Once you know some sign language, try to carry on a conversation using only sign. Notice how graceful it can be. The National Theatre for the Deaf in Waterford, Connecticut, has given performances all around the country. Sign language as well as verbal communication is used. Try to go to see a live performance. You will have an opportunity to view sign done in a highly creative fashion.

## FINGERSPELLING

There are hand positions for every letter of the alphabet in fingerspelling. Practice making the letters. Once you feel

[53

# FINGER SPELLING
## as seen by the viewer

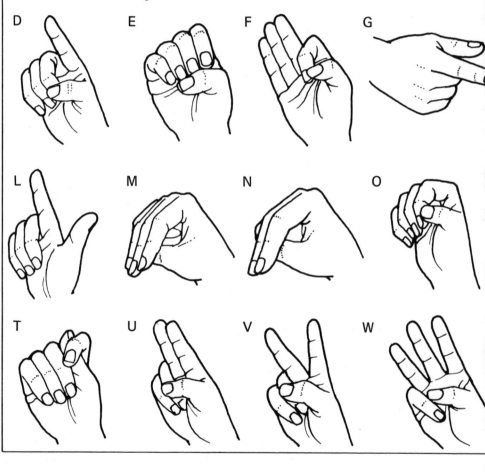

D E F G

L M N O

T U V W

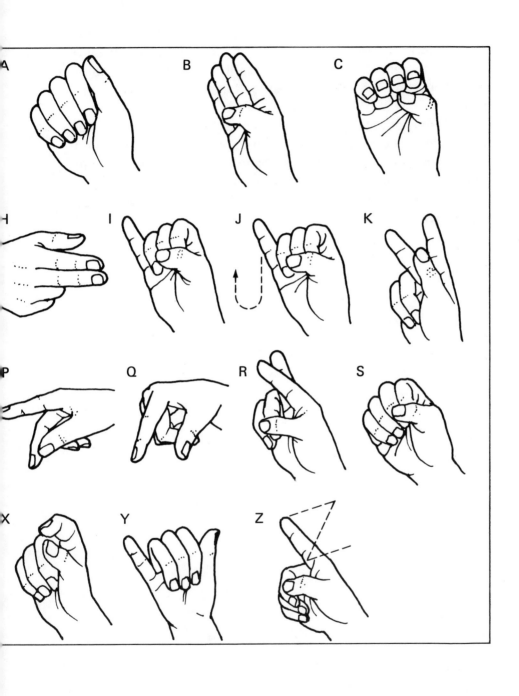

you can form the letters, try to use fingerspelling to convey a message to someone. How long does it take? Can you understand fingerspelling when someone "talks" to you using their hands?

Hearing people can only try to imagine what it is like not to be able to hear well. Some of the things you may have tried might have been fun. Some may have been harder to do than others. Try to imagine what it would be like to communicate using some of these techniques all of the time. What if you didn't have a choice?

# Glossary

Audiologist—a specially trained person who tests one's ability to hear.

Audiometer—an instrument often used by an audiologist to measure a person's ability to hear.

Auditory Method—one of the methods used to teach speech and language to the hearing-impaired child. This method requires the student to concentrate on developing listening skills. It is often used with children who have a moderate hearing loss.

Auditory nerve—the path along which the chemical electrical energy produced in the inner ear is sent to the brain.

Bilateral hearing loss—a hearing loss involving both ears.

[57

Cochlea—a part of the inner ear that contains very small sensory cells surrounded by fluid. The motion of this fluid causes a chemical electrical impulse that is then passed to the brain by way of the auditory nerve.

Conductive hearing loss—usually a temporary hearing loss often due to an infection, buildup of wax, or injury to the ear.

Decibel (db)—a measure of sound's intensity.

External ear canal—a short tunnel between the outer ear and the eardrum.

Fingerspelling—a method of communication that uses various finger positions for each letter of the alphabet.

Incus—one of the three tiny bones in the middle ear that help conduct sound waves from the eardrum to the inner ear; also called the anvil.

Inner ear—a fluid-filled cavity that contains the cochlea, the organ responsible for balance.

Malleus—one of three tiny bones in the middle ear that help conduct sound waves from the eardrum to the inner ear; also called the hammer.

Middle ear—the air-filled space located behind the eardrum. It contains three bones (malleus, incus, and stapes) that conduct sound waves from the eardrum to the inner ear.

Oral Method—one of the methods used to teach speech and language to the hearing-impaired child. The student learns through speech reading or lipreading and often makes use of a hearing aid.

Ossicles—name given collectively to all three bones contained in the middle ear (malleus, incus, and stapes).

Outer ear—refers to the pinna (or auricle), the external ear canal, and the eardrum (or tympanic membrane).

Oval and Round Windows—somewhat transparent windows that separate the middle and inner ear.

Pinna—the visible portion of the ear, the pinna funnels incoming sound waves into the external ear canal; also called the auricle.

Rochester Method—one of the methods used to teach speech and language to the hearing-impaired child. It combines the oral method with fingerspelling.

Sensorineural Hearing Loss—a permanent loss caused by damage to the sensory cells. These hearing losses may get worse over time.

Sign Language—a method of communication using the hands and arms to represent a particular thought. Facial expressions and body postures are also used to convey meanings.

Simultaneous Method—one of the methods used to teach speech and language to the hearing-impaired child. It is a combination of the oral method, sign language, and fingerspelling.

Stapes—one of three tiny bones in the middle ear that help conduct sound waves from the eardrum to the inner ear. Also called the stirrup.

Temporal Lobes—that part of the brain which receives most of the messages connected with hearing.

Total Communication—one of the methods used to teach speech and language to the hearing-impaired child. This method encourages the use of all forms of communication, including speech, gestures, pantomime, fingerspelling, and sign language.

Tympanic membrane—contained in the outer ear, sound waves strike this membrane, and cause it to vibrate; also called the eardrum.

# For Further Reading

Brown, Marion Marsh, and Crone, Ruth. *The Silent Storm.* Nashville: Abingdon Press, 1963.

Charlip, Remy, and Miller, Mary Beth, and Ancona, George. *Hand Talk, An ABC of Finger Spelling and Sign Language.* New York: Parents' Magazine Press, 1974.

Graff, Stewart, and Polly Anne. *Helen Keller—Toward the Light.* Champaign: Garrard Publishing Co., 1965.

Hunter, Edith Fisher. *Child of the Silent Night.* Boston: Houghton Mifflin, 1963.

Keller, Helen Adams. *The Story of My Life.* New York: Doubleday & Co., 1903.

Litchfield, Ada B. *A Button in Her Ear.* Chicago: Albert Whitman & Co., 1976.

Peare, Catherine Owens. *The Helen Keller Story*. New York: Thomas Y. Crowell Co., Inc., 1959.

Peterson, Jeanne Whitehouse. *I Have a Sister, My Sister Is Deaf*. New York: Harper & Row, 1977.

Robinson, Veronica. *David in Silence*. Philadelphia: J. P. Lippincott Co., 1965.

# Index